12 LEAPS OF FAITH TO BECOME A TRAVEL NURSE

The Ultimate Step-by-Step Guide

Amber Black

Ebook ISBN: 978-0-578-35278-7
Paperback ISBN: 978-0-578-35277-0

Edited by Amber Black & Amanda Callisaya
Cover Art by Amber Black & Pro_EbookCovers
Layout by Amber Black
Author Photograph by Courtney Truly

First edition published and printed in the USA

AVB Publishing
Selma, AL

Library of Congress Control Number: 2022900177

For information or permission requests contact:
amber.black14@gmail.com

Dedication

I dedicate this book to all my nurses and nursing students who aspire to travel but do not know where to start. Whether you are from a small town like me or a big city, I designed this travel nursing guide to make your transition as easy and efficient as possible. It includes my personal experiences in hopes that they can help you avoid some of my mistakes. Here's to you, because I believe you can do this too!

Table of Contents

Introduction

Travel nursing is a profession that helps to fill the need for temporary staffing in healthcare facilities. Travel nurses may work for multiple organizations and are usually "on assignment" or contracted for weeks at a time. There are many tiers to travel nursing such as local, national, and international. This guide is catered more towards the national aspect of travel nursing, as state-to-state is the most common type. However, these steps can guide you in the right direction to start local or international travel nursing as well. Whether you are a current travel nurse, a staff nurse aspiring to travel, or a nursing student, this guide is comprehensive and may contain information you will find useful for years to come.

Travel nursing is beneficial because the money is good—BIG BAG! But seriously, all jokes aside, travel nurses are in demand due to nursing shortages, and will continue to be in the foreseeable future. In addition to job security, the benefits of travel nursing include exploring new places, avoiding workplace politics, flexibility, and career advancement opportunities, just to name a few. Most importantly, wherever you decide to go, you are helping a facility that is in desperate need and touching the lives of more patients as a travel nurse.

Is travel nursing right for you? This is a question you have to ask yourself. If you are reading this book then obviously you have some sort of interest in this billion-dollar industry. So before we get started, I would like to highlight a few key points. Everyone comes from different backgrounds. What one person may deem difficult, another person may classify as easy. Don't compare yourself and don't scare yourself! The more prepared you are prior to your travel nursing journey, the more likely you are to have good outcomes. I am here to help you figure it all out, so let's get right into it!

Step 1: Obtain a Nursing Degree ✓

First things first, you need a nursing degree. A 4-year Bachelor of Science in Nursing (BSN) is preferable, but another option is a 2-year Associate of Science in Nursing (ASN). I chose to go to Troy University right after high school. However, some people pursue nursing later in life and that's fine too! To begin, research colleges nearby, apply for scholarships, take prerequisites, and get accepted into a nursing program. Nursing school is not easy. It requires a lot of time and discipline, but you can do it. Just be prepared for studying and clinicals. Clinicals are supervised patient interactions designed to facilitate learning.

This is also the point where you should obtain your BLS certification through your nursing program. BLS stands for basic life support and is a mandatory certification to work in healthcare. You will be renewing this certification every two years for the rest of your nursing career. It's great to get it issued and out the way now. If your nursing program is not offering BLS certifications, look for resources provided by the American Heart Association in surrounding areas.

You can begin applying and interviewing for nursing jobs as a new graduate RN during your last semester of nursing school. Your actual job acceptance to start work will still depend on completion of your nursing program and passing the NCLEX, unless you file for a temporary work permit.

Step 2: Pass the NCLEX to Receive Home State RN License ✓

The NCLEX, or National Council Licensure Exam, is a nationwide, standardized test that every nursing student must pass post-graduation to receive their RN license to be eligible to work. It is the state's way of verifying your knowledge. The test itself costs $200 and consists of 75–265 questions of nursing content from various categories. The number of questions a test-taker will have to answer varies because of the way the test is designed. The questions are primarily multiple-choice, but are not limited to this. You have a maximum of six hours to complete the exam, and receive your results in about 48 hours. I always suggest taking it as soon as possible after nursing school, while the content is still fresh in your mind. You can utilize any study material you find helpful, but I personally used HURST Review. I took the exam approximately four weeks after graduation and passed on the first try. That said, I studied for about two weeks straight prior to test day. I did not go anywhere or do anything but study 5–8 hours a day and relax afterwards. The NCLEX was my only focus. I had a little strategy of studying by body systems. Yes, I was nervous…all the way up until receiving my results. Trust yourself because like the saying goes, "Being nervous isn't bad, it just means something important is happening." If you happen to fail, that is okay. I highly encourage you to RE-TEST! You got this!

Step 3: Gain 2 Years of Work Experience ✓

I would suggest that you pick one field/specialty to go into post-graduation and stick with it for two years. Why? Because you need all of this time to become competent in tasks, charting, and critical thinking. I started in the NICU (Neonatal Intensive Care Unit) as a new graduate at Children's of Alabama in 2018, and I am now a NICU travel nurse. For the most part, I always knew I wanted to be a NICU nurse. Luckily that unit welcomed new grads with open arms, because not every facility/specialty hires new grads in the unit. I am sure you've heard a lot of people say that new grads have to start in "med-surg"—well that is not true. (Med-surg is what we like to call the Medical-Surgical Unit.) If you know what area you want to pursue, try researching or asking around about facilities that welcome new grads into specialties so you can gain that experience right away.

Healthcare facilities do not just look at your overall years of experience as a nurse, but also how long you were in the specialty that you are applying for as a travel nurse. For example, facilities looking to hire NICU travel nurses may be more inclined to choose my application, since I have been a NICU nurse for three years, over that of another nurse who has five years of nursing experience but only eight months in the NICU. Does that make sense? Two years of experience is not required but it is preferred amongst most facilities when hiring travel nurses. Some facilities are more lenient and will accept a minimum of six months experience.

Some new nurses are unsure of which area they will like, so they go from unit to unit at first and that is okay. Once you find your happy place, gain as much experience as possible there before applying as a travel nurse. Also, while you are there gaining experience, it would be beneficial to utilize the facility's free resources for obtaining additional unit-specific certifications (ACLS, NRP, STABLE, PALS, etc.) right before resigning. However, you may also wait until step 9 to do so through your agency.

Step 4: Research and Apply with Travel Nursing Agencies to Build a Profile ✓

DO YOUR RESEARCH! There are hundreds of travel nursing agencies out there and not all with the intentions of doing their absolute best for YOU as the client. When I started applying to agencies, I went strictly based on recommendations from close friends who had travel nursing experience. Even then, you still want to research those agencies to see if they fit your needs, have good benefits (medical, vision, dental, 401k, life insurance), sick pay, license and travel reimbursements, etc. I suggest that you apply to 2–4 agencies at a time and build your profiles. Why? Because it's good to have options. Every agency pays out differently and has different benefits, so it is nice to compare. It is also free to apply and betters your chances of landing a contract with high pay rates. For example, multiple agencies have access to the same assignment, but one may offer more money. Having multiple agencies under your belt leaves room for negotiating and increases your knowledge in the travel nursing market.

However, some may find duplicating information to multiple agencies to be overwhelming or annoying. To date, I have changed agencies three times. But I've stayed with my current agency for the past nine months because it is convenient. I still have profiles with other agencies that I occasionally update when it is time to relocate, just to compare numbers. So at the end of the day, when it comes down to choosing agencies, do what works best for you.

When you join an agency, you will be given a recruiter. Your recruiter is usually randomly assigned to you, unless you ask for someone specifically by name. They are your point of contact within the agency to help you with EVERYTHING. It is important to make sure that the two of you are bonding and have a good working relationship. Some recruiters are chill and helpful, and others can be rude or annoying. Your recruiter should listen to your preferences and get you the most money possible. If they are argumentative, "ghost" you, guilt-trip you, or try to pressure you in decision-making, then they're fired! (Maybe not literally by the agency, but definitely by YOU.) You can simply request for someone else within the agency or move on completely to a different agency and recruiter. You, your agency, and your recruiter should work together as a team.

While building your profile, which is much like a resume, you will need your pertinent work history, education history, licenses, certifications, references, and complete a skills checklist. It is imperative to complete your profile ASAP! Doing so will give you a jumpstart advantage to landing a contract and lessen your chances of missing out on an opportunity. Most profiles can be completed in a few hours.

Step 5: Obtain Desired State's Nursing License ✓

If you are planning to travel to a different state, you will need an active nursing license in that state. Do not worry, your recruiter can help with this part. Hopefully, your home state is a part of the Nurse Licensure Compact (NLC). If they are, then you can simply pay for a multi-state license. The NLC is an agreement between some states that allows nurses to have one license, with the ability to practice in all states that are part of the agreement. As of July 6th, 2021, there are 37 states and one territory that are included in the NLC. However, if either your home state or the state you want to travel to is NOT within the compact, then you must apply and pay for a nursing license in your desired state. For example, my home state is Alabama. Alabama joined the NLC in 2020. I immediately applied for the multi-state license and it was issued within the same week (I say "applied" because that's what the board of nursing calls it, but you're really just filling out basic personal information and paying hundreds of dollars, ha!) Georgia is also a part of the NLC, so I decided to go there for my first contract, not too far from home. However, when I finally decided to go to California, which is NOT a part of the NLC, I had to apply for a nursing license by endorsement with the California Board of Nursing. I had to pay about $300 and wait three months for it to be processed and issued. The California BON is very slow, so if you are applying there, please expect a long wait and plan ahead.

Unfortunately, if your home state is currently not a part of the compact, you must obtain a single state license by endorsement for every state you wish to travel to. Licenses from other states that are not a part of the compact may also be obtained via "fast-track," but only if it is offered. Otherwise it may take anywhere from as little as a few days to as long as a few months. Another option would be filing for a temporary license to work while you wait on the permanent license by endorsement. During times of a "crisis," like COVID-19, states may temporarily allow outside nurses to work in their state without having that state's license at all. Your recruiter will notify you of any fast-track or crisis situations.

Step 6: Browse and Submit to Job Openings ✓

Once your profile is complete and you have your nursing license for whatever state you want to travel to, the job hunt begins! You and your recruiter will work together to find the best assignment for you. Travel nursing is much like Burger King. You can have it your way—at least most of the time. Tell your recruiter what city you want to be in, approximately how much you want to get paid, what shift you prefer, etc. Of course, you may not always get everything, but express all your preferences anyway. Sometimes you may have to compromise just a little, so it is important to be flexible. Just know what is non-negotiable for you! Personally, I will only work the night shift and (3) 12-hour shifts per week. If nothing is available in the area at the time, I will wait it out or go elsewhere.

You will review job requirements and pay packages during this part of the process. Requirements will include work experience, certifications, and more. The pay package is probably the most important topic, right? Well if you aren't budgeting already, now is a good time to start. You need to know how much your bills and other expenses are going to cost you monthly during this chapter in your life. Why? Because budgeting can help you decide how much money you're willing to accept on a contract—after all, you want to make a profit, not break even!

Pay packages vary by state, specialty/unit, and agency. Almost any contract is more money than what you would make as a staff nurse. The pay is a huge factor in why someone becomes a travel nurse, plus the traveling experience. As a travel nurse in the state of Georgia, I was making double what I was as a staff nurse in Alabama—now I am making 7x that in California. You can easily make six figures in less than a year as a travel nurse. I have seen contracts anywhere from $1,000–$10,000+ PER WEEK! Of course, this spike has a lot to do with the COVID-19 pandemic, but even before that, travel nurses still made good money.

As a travel nurse, you will get paid weekly your hourly rate, which is taxed, plus tax-free housing/meal stipends. However, you can only collect tax-free stipends if you meet requirements set by the IRS. This brings me back to those tiers of nursing I mentioned in the intro (local, national, international). I highly recommend speaking with a tax specialist or CPA to help you understand what is or is not legally appropriate to collect as a local, national, or international travel nurse. If you do not abide by the laws of the IRS, you put yourself at risk of owing back taxes on the stipend money that you received or paying a huge fine. It may even cost you your freedom. Therefore, a major resource that has been helpful to many travel nurses is traveltax.com.

If you are only given a summarized pay package, be sure to request an itemized breakdown—this goes into more detail so you can calculate things yourself. Paycheckcity.com is a website that travel nurses like to use to determine their potential take-home after taxes. The itemized pay package will include: regular hourly rate, overtime rate, stipends, holiday rate, on call/call back rate, travel bonus/allowance, and estimated gross/net. Make sure your stipends will actually cover your housing needs. I quickly realized rent in California definitely weren't those Alabama prices, ha! Please expect pay rates to correspond with the level of the market. But honey, let me tell you—when facilities are in great need, the market is booming with hourly rates as high as $100+.

(Side note: In California, you get paid a certain amount for the first 8 hours of work, known as a regular hourly rate. Then you are paid an "overtime" amount for the last 4 hours of a 12-hour shift. I talk about California a lot because that is usually where the best contracts, weather, and experiences are and that is where I have been working for over a year now. To give you an example of Southern California contracts, I once took an offer for $3,800/week take-home—that is good for NICU.)

After reviewing pay packages, it is time to submit. Submit means that your recruiter electronically shoots your profile over to the facility as a candidate for the posted assignment. You may submit your profile to multiple facilities that spark your interest. (If by any chance you are missing a requirement, such as a certification, do not hesitate to submit. Facilities may still offer you the position as long as you agree to obtain the certification, etc. by your start date.) The whole submission process can roll pretty fast, so be ready. Once you tell your recruiter to submit you to a job opening, you can hear back as early as the same day with an offer. However, since the market has become more saturated and competitive in recent years, some assignments may take up to two weeks to fill. Within your submission, be sure to include your desired start date. Facilities hire anywhere from immediate start to four weeks out max, so there is no need to browse openings and submit 2-3 months before you are even ready to start. They will reject your profile until time gets closer. You also need to provide any requests for time off. Requested time off is usually approved with a limit of about 5-7 days. (I always request a week off every contract, because why not take a vacation or staycation? But you do not get paid for RTO. In order for me to still get all of my contracted hours in, I take off Wednesday–Tuesday, instead of the traditional Sunday–Saturday. That way I can still work 36 hours the week of and after my vacation.) Then when all this is done, wait patiently on feedback from your recruiter in regards to an interview, automatic offer, or position-filled status.

Step 7: Prepare For Interviews ✓

Managers may call you for a phone interview, or the process may be all virtual. I know a lot of us nurses, especially on night shift, like to keep our phones on "Do Not Disturb" when we are sleeping during the daytime, but you do not want to miss that interview call. Keep your phone on at all times during this waiting period, because managers may or may not ask for a specific date/time to contact you. If you happen to miss the call though, do not fret, my friend! They should leave a voicemail with instructions for you to call them back. Always present yourself in a positive light. Even negative work experiences can be used to your advantage. Smile, be authentic and confident. Show them you are trustworthy as a travel nurse, because safety is always important. Jot down unique qualities that make you stand out, along with skills you are competent in. The following are common questions you should ask at the end of the interview:

1. What charting system is used? (Epic, Cerner, Meditech, etc.)
2. How many beds are on the unit? What are the nurse-to-patient ratios and census normally like? (You want to know what you're walking into…busy unit = less floating).
3. What is the scrub color for nurses?

4. When can I expect to hear back?

Virtual interviews mean you answer interview questions online with written and voice-recorded responses. Sometimes you are offered the position and do not have an interview at all. I like those the best, ha! This is known as the automatic or "auto offer" I mentioned earlier. If you get an auto offer, but have questions for the manager about the unit, you can still call on your own prior to your start date. Your recruiter can provide the manager's contact information.

Step 8: Review Offer/Contract and Sign or Decline ✓

If the facility likes what they see on your profile, they will send an offer to your recruiter. Your recruiter will then notify you of the great news. A formal contract will be sent to you for your review. A travel nursing contract is essentially a written agreement between the nurse, an agency, and the facility. Contracts explain specific terms and conditions that all parties must abide by. Each contract's verbiage is different, but it is your sole responsibility to make sure everything is correct and in your best interest.

Terms usually mentioned in a contract are start date, location of facility, float requirements, shift, hours per week, length of assignment, attendance/cancellation policy, requested time off, and pay. Review it carefully and make sure it is precise. We are all human and people can make mistakes. Once you are comfortable with the numbers and policies, you will sign electronically and you officially have an assignment. YAY! Go celebrate, because I sure as hell did the first time—and every time thereafter. (Let's face it, I don't need much of an excuse to go out partying with my friends anyway, ha!)

Because I am not the type to have all my eggs in one basket, I would suggest keeping your current job up until this exact point of signing. Then you can put in a notice for your resignation or see about dropping down to PRN/as needed or per diem status. Hopefully, you already made your current manager somewhat aware that you were looking into travel nursing, so that it's not a complete shock.

On the other end of the spectrum, you have the decision to decline an offer. You may choose to decline due to personal obligations that come up, or because you already received a better offer elsewhere. Whatever the case may be, just be cautious of declining offers you interviewed for. This can be frowned upon. Yes, we take that chance when submitting to multiple facilities at once, but just be mindful during this process. Essentially, you should only submit to an assignment you're willing to accept. The best thing to do when submitting to multiple facilities is to have your recruiter retract your profile from the other submissions once your first offer rolls in. Retracting removes your profile from the candidate pool, which is different from declining an offer. In some circumstances, when you would rather wait to hear back from a higher paying submission, you can politely request 24 hours to think about the first offer you've been given. This gives the higher paying facility more time to respond without you completely giving up on an opportunity. Whether or not the higher paying facility responds within 24 hours, you will still need to make a decision: decline and wait, or accept and begin onboarding.

Step 9: Begin Onboarding Process ✓

Onboarding is defined as the steps you need to complete prior to your start date. Travel nurses go through an onboarding process with every new assignment, but the steps may vary. A few days after signing you should receive an email from your recruiter (or their colleague in the Compliance Department, also known as a credentialing specialist) with all the information the facility needs from you to start. These things include lab work, documents/certifications, and tests. The lab work required by most facilities includes a flu vaccine, urine drug screen, physical and vision exam, mask fit test, TB skin test, and titers or immunizations/boosters for MMR, Varicella, Hep B, etc. If you already have these health records, GREAT—send in a copy. If not, your agency will find a nearby clinic for you to get everything done at no cost to you. Documents such as your driver's license, social security card, nursing license, direct deposit information, proof of permanent home address, W-4 and I-9 tax documents, questionnaires, attestations, and other policy agreement forms requiring your personal information and electronic signature may be requested. As previously stated, I suggest getting your basic certifications back in step 3 to cut down on this already lengthy onboarding process. However, if any additional certifications are required by the facility, now is the time to get them. Your agency can help you find a nearby provider and reimburse you.

Next, you have lengthy and seemingly unnecessary online exams, such as Prophecy Health Exams called "RN Core Mandatory" or comparable competency exams. Pharmacology and/or arrhythmia exams are common, as well as unit-specific modules via Healthstream or a similar platform. Try not to stress too much about these, because most answers are common sense or can be found on the World Wide Web. Nonetheless, remember that this step is very time-consuming. Your facility may also require some online training on their charting system before starting. There will be a deadline for everything, so do not get behind!

Step 10: Find Housing and Prepare to Move ✓

FurnishedFinder.com is my go-to for housing. You get to bypass those ridiculous fees that are on Airbnb and other sites. Otherwise, creating an account and using FurnishedFinder is very similar to how Airbnb operates. It is super user-friendly, and even has an app you can download, though I prefer using the browser. You can filter or sort listings down to your liking and save them in your Favorites to view later. You can message hosts on the website or via the contact number/email that is provided. There are pictures, reviews, descriptions, and a map. FurnishedFinder is geared towards extended stays of one month or longer, which is perfect for us travel nurses. Its rentals are obviously furnished, hence the name, and utilities are included. Some hosts may request a formal rental application and background check. Next, you discuss accommodations and payment methods with the host, but be sure to get it in writing along with monthly rental receipts for your records. Since contracts can be canceled, it is important to mention this to your host so that there won't be any problems getting your deposit and/or first month's rent back—even a prorated refund should be feasible. I never had any issues with housing. But of course, there is always a chance things are not as they seem online. So just be careful and do not be afraid to speak up, ask questions, or request more pictures/videos. If you are in the area, go check it out in person. It is also a good idea to research the general area for leisure activities, safety, and essentials.

Some hosts rent out private homes, guest houses, studios, or apartments. Others rent out bedrooms in a shared home with private or shared bathrooms and common areas. I have experienced them all and must say I prefer studio-styles because it is the cheapest, private option. Making a list of non-negotiables might help with your search. My must-have list for housing is: A/C and heating, kitchen, private bathroom, parking, and WiFi. I also like to be no more than 30 minutes from work. Other things like washer/dryer and television I can compromise on, especially since staying within my budget is most important to me. There is always a laundromat nearby. I can always buy and resell a cheap TV.

Other housing resources to consider are Facebook groups (Gypsy Nursing), VRBO, and the previously mentioned Airbnb. Most hotels and suites/extended stays have discounted rates for healthcare workers (but it ain't enough of a discount for me, ha!). RVs are another common form of housing (and transportation) in the travel nursing world. Your agency can also find you housing but it is more expensive—we're trying to maximize our profit around here, okay! Whichever route you take, be sure to speak with the host directly. Let them know you are a travel nurse and always ask for a lower price than what is listed, it won't hurt to try.

Whether or not you are keeping your primary house/apartment is an important thing to consider. I gave up pretty much everything to save the most money as a travel nurse. Vacating my first apartment as an adult was bittersweet—after all, I had been there for two years and really loved that place—but I did not want to pay rent in two different places, eating my freaking check. Giving up my previous place also meant I had no utility bill, internet bill, etc. I sold some furniture, small appliances, household items, and clothes/shoes. Then I packed up what I wanted to keep into two separate piles: what was going into storage and what was coming with me. I rented a 10x10 controlled storage unit for $100 in a safe area (which I still have to this day). Also, do not forget to discontinue your utilities and sign up for mail forwarding. I filed for my mail to be forwarded to my parents' home for one year for free via USPS. I also get a PO Box everywhere I go for online shopping purposes.

If you have been following my journey, you may know I decided to take that 2,000 mile, 3-day road trip from Alabama to California. I only spent about $600 doing so (on hotels, gas, and food) versus getting my SUV shipped for $1,000. I just felt like driving was cheaper and less of a hassle, plus I have a lot of stuff. I have a few travel nurse friends who prefer the latter, though. Choose what works best for you. Just as an insight, my friend and I started at sunrise on a Friday and took turns driving my loaded-down car 5 hours per person, per day. We made it to my destination on that following Sunday. You can really make it fun if you choose to drive across the country.

If you choose not to take a car at all, you can utilize public transportation in bigger cities or even get a rental there—I hear Turo is pretty affordable. If you are flying to your destination, definitely limit your belongings to only a few suitcases, because that's $30+ per checked bag depending on the airline. You could also choose to ship boxes of your belongings. I have used UPS and it was affordable and fast. With all that being said, I am not going to list out my recommendations on what exactly you should take with you, because I pack entirely too much, ha! It is very easy to accumulate things overtime. Pack what you regularly use and perhaps buy more as needs present themselves—just don't forget your scrubs.

Step 11: Follow First Day Instructions for Orientation ✓

After you are cleared from the onboarding process, you will receive an email of "First Day Instructions" from your recruiter. It will likely give you an itinerary, parking details, dress code, badge information, timekeeping, and more. You may be required to complete even more online modules on-site before working with a preceptor. Orientation is typically a total of only 1-3 days. Then you hit the ball rolling on your own! So take down any notes you may need, like door codes, etc.

At this point you may be nervous. As stated before, that can be expected a lot in life. You're going to do great and everything is going to be fine. I am sure you are a great nurse or you would not have made it this far. Have some confidence to help ease some of your fear. But remember, you never want to be too comfortable or "too good" to adapt to change or receive constructive criticism. Every facility runs differently. Go in with a smile, ready to work, and after your first few weeks, you will feel like a part of the team.

If anything unexpected happens, just notify your recruiter. Always remember, this is your license that you worked hard for that's on the line. If you are uncomfortable at any point, do not be afraid to speak up. You are allowed to refuse a patient assignment if you feel that it is unsafe for you or the patients. You must refuse prior to taking report, or handoff, on the patients. If you take report and then choose to walk away from the assignment, that is considered abandonment.

Step 12: Extend Contract or Repeat Steps #4-11 for Next Assignment ✓

Thirteen weeks, or however long you are contracted for, will fly by! If you really like it at that facility, at any point you can tell your recruiter, "Hey, I want to request an extension." Sometimes the facilities ask you first. It also doesn't hurt to ask for a raise with the extension.

However, if you are ready to move on, go ahead and start thinking about your next game plan towards the end of your current contract. You can also choose to take a break for however long you decide. Maybe you want to be off for two months to enjoy the winter holidays or summer sun. I, personally, take breaks of anywhere from 2–4 weeks in between assignments. Once I decide on the date I want to start working again, I notify my recruiter (or find a new agency) of this new potential start date. Together, we start browsing again 3–4 weeks out from my chosen date. Just the thought of not having any job secured makes me a little anxious. I don't like to wait until the last minute. That way I have time to rest, relocate, do onboarding, etc.

Before you know it, you will feel like a seasoned travel nurse. To date, I have been a NICU travel nurse for 1.5 years and completed 4 assignments. I truly hope you take that leap of faith to start your journey as a travel nurse, and that my guide provides some help along the way. I used to be where you are now. I was clueless and only knew a few people who could lead me in the right direction (big shoutout to my girl Halle Berry). My sole purpose in writing this guide is to be that helping hand for you. The whole process and thought of traveling may seem scary or hard at first, but it gets easier. You may be thinking, "I'm about to quit my staff job, sign my life over in this contract, get rid of my apartment, go across the country where I know no one, to be a travel nurse"—trust me, I've been there. But I can almost guarantee you will love this career path. It has been the best decision I have made. Although not every assignment may be perfect, all the good experiences will outweigh the bad. You will learn new things at work and experience new things on your days off. Not to mention, you will meet a ton of new people, all while making some really good money. Lastly, stay safe out there y'all—especially the brave, solo travel nurses like myself. You got this. I believe all things will work together for your good. Now that you have all the information, I guess it is up to you to decide…Are you ready to take ***12 leaps of faith*** to become a profitable travel nurse?

Frequently Asked Questions

1. **What types of patients will I get as a travel nurse?**

   This varies at each facility; some are more lenient than others when assigning to travelers. But it is not uncommon for travelers to receive the "worst assignment" or heavier workload. I have been there and persevered—so will you. You can do anything for 13 weeks friend, cha-ching!

2. **Can I become a travel nurse as a new grad?**

   Most facilities require 6 months to 1 year minimum experience, but preferably 2 years.

3. **What is "blacklisting," or "DNR"?**

   Blacklisting in the nursing world is essentially being boycotted from a facility, chain, or agency. This can be due to canceling your contract, safety concerns, etc. DNR stands for Do Not Return.

4. **Can my contract get canceled?**

   Yes, a contract can be canceled at any time by you or the facility. Most contracts are in agreement to "at-will employment." This means either party may terminate the contract at any moment, resulting in a dismissal of any fulfillment duties remaining. If a facility does cancel, your recruiter will notify you. Simply repeat the steps to find a new assignment. Inform your recruiter if you need to cancel a contract for whatever reason.

5. **Will travel nurses always be in demand?**

   In my opinion, yes, because healthcare is forever and nursing shortages are actually increasing due to COVID-19, nurse retirements, birth rates, and other contributing factors. Travel nursing has been around for decades.

6. **How do I file taxes as a travel nurse?**

   I suggest using a tax professional for help.

7. **What are some recommended agencies?**

   So far I have worked with Medical Solutions, Talemed (which has now combined with Triage), and Emerald Health Services. Other agencies with good standing are Travel Nurses Across America, Aya, Atlas, and Trustaff. Agencies with a reputation of high paying rates are American Mobile Network, Krucial Staffing, and Maxim Health. Agencies known for international contracts are Ventura Medstaff, Travel PHP, and Alium Consultancy.

8. **Can I travel with a family and pets?**

   Yes, but pet fees may apply for housing.

9. **How far in advance do I apply to agencies?**

   Apply to agencies when you are ready to take that leap as a travel nurse. As soon as your profile is built, you can submit to openings. The process rolls pretty fast after that.

10. **How long are assignments?**

Assignments can be anywhere from 4 – 14 weeks initially. You may have the option to extend longer.

11. Can I choose where I go?

Yes. However, if no assignments are available at that time in your preferred location, you may want to look elsewhere.

12. Can I take off or call out sick as a travel nurse?

You can submit time off in advance in your contract for vacations, etc. After that, callouts/missed shifts will simply not be paid, along with some of the stipend for that week. However, some agencies do let you accrue sick time. Please call out per policy, which is usually 2 hours before start of shift. No call no show is frowned upon.

13. What's the best shift to work as a travel nurse?

The best shift to work as a travel nurse is strictly your preference. I suggest you go with what you were used to working as staff, unless you deem otherwise. You can choose from days, nights, or rotating. Most contracts are written for 12 hour shifts (7a/p – 7p/a, 3 days a week or 36 hrs). Some facilities may offer more or less days/hours depending on their needs.

14. Are staff nurses really rude to travel nurses?

Most facilities are very travel-friendly, but you will always have a few that are not as accepting. Staff nurses tend not to understand the bigger picture: we are here to fill the needs where their unit lacks. I hope embracing travelers becomes the norm at EVERY facility in the near future

15. Will I be scheduled to work every weekend as a travel nurse?

Not necessarily. Some facilities allow travelers to self-schedule along with their staff, while others place you where needed. If you are expected to work every weekend that is usually presented when applying. One weekend a month or every other weekend are common requirements you may see as well.

Sample Interview Questions

1. What are your strengths/weaknesses?
2. What would you do in _____ situation and how would you overcome it?
3. How do you provide exceptional customer service?
4. Why are you interested in being a travel nurse here?
5. Why should we hire you?
6. What has been your biggest conflict in the workplace?
7. How do you handle stress?
8. Are you comfortable and willing to float?
9. Think of a difficult time when you dealt with an angry patient or their family member. How did you handle it?
10. What types of patients have you taken care of?
11. You have been assigned a patient admitted on the previous shift for possible _____. Explain what it is and the signs and symptoms you might expect.

Questions to Ask During Orientation

1. What needs to be documented and how often?
2. Are doctors/NPs, RTs, techs, and clerks on site 24/7 and how do I reach them?
3. What is the manager's name and phone number?
4. What is the facility and unit phone number?
5. How do I reach lab and pharmacy?
6. Is the cafeteria open late? (lunch/snacks are important too, especially for night shift)
7. Who do I contact for scheduling?
8. Where can I find the unit policies and procedures?
9. What is your code and procedure for emergencies?

Helpful Tips

- ✓ Periodically update your profile with your favorite agencies.
- ✓ Be organized. Save health records, documents, license/certifications, onboarding tests, and interview questions/responses in one place for easier access.
- ✓ Have everything in writing. This includes whatever "promises" your agency or facility verbally makes (ex. reimbursements). A simple email will suffice.
- ✓ Build rapport with some of the staff nurses, managers, and/or charge nurses. Not only will you need a reference later, but having a helping hand from someone more familiar with the unit is nice too.
- ✓ Do not be afraid to ask doctors, nursing staff, or techs questions whenever you are not sure about something.
- ✓ Travelers often stick together by helping one another with patient care, offering advice, or giving insight on a facility. They tend to make great hangout buddies outside of work as well. We are like our own community, so make friends.
- ✓ Take advantage of "strikes."
- ✓ Consider joining the following Facebook groups: Travel Nurse Jobs $5000 a Week and Up, Crisis Rates Nursing Jobs, Travel Nursing: The Premium Job Board, Short-term/Per Diem Travel Nurse Assignments Nationwide, Travel Nurse Housing – The Gypsy Nurse, Travel Nursing: Places/Rooms for Rent, Travel Nursing Newbies, Travel Nursing: The $4000 and Up Club,

Travel Nurse Housing – Furnished Finder, and Team Healthcare Strike

- ✓ Search travel nursing FB groups according to your specialty. For my fellow NICU nurses, here's a few: NICU Travel Nursing Jobs, NICU Nurses & Travel Nurses (not Recruiters), and Premium NICU Travel Assignments
- ✓ Do not get involved in unit drama.
- ✓ Do things their way to avoid confusion.
- ✓ Do not discuss your pay with staff. We are here to take care of the patient, mind our business, and get to the bag—in and out, sis!
- ✓ Most travel nurses work with multiple agencies; it is okay to submit your profile to different facilities through the same agency. However, try to avoid submitting your profile to the same facility under different agencies.
- ✓ Only float to areas of competency. For example, as a NICU nurse if I float to PICU/Peds I will only accept patients 2 years old or younger. If I float to an adult floor, I am only assisting as a runner or secretary. Be sure to specify this in your contract.
- ✓ Become travel nurses with a buddy. It is probably more fun that way and makes things like housing a lot cheaper.
- ✓ Stay on top of re-certifications—usually every 2 years.
- ✓ Know what you can and cannot do as a nurse. Each facility/state has different rules or laws for nurses. For example, some facilities allow nurses to put in orders and draw labs, while others do not.
- ✓ Don't talk too much about what facilities you've been to, where you're going next, or where you're living— this

goes for both staff nurses and social media outlets. Some people have ulterior motives or hidden agendas.

- ✓ Maintain an active status for each state's nursing license you have by renewing on time every 2 years. Online renewal (and CEU requirements) are required if you want to continue to work there or plan to go back there in the near future.
- ✓ Save about $2–4k before applying as a traveler. You will need this money for travel expenses and to secure housing. (You will not get your first paycheck as a travel nurse until the second week of work). Unexpected things come along with the territory of travel nursing, so it is important to be prepared with an emergency fund.
- ✓ Do not be afraid to speak up when negotiating contracts. The worst they can say is NO! But then you will just move on to the next opportunity because everything happens for a reason. But what if they say YES? See, closed mouths don't get fed boo, ha!

Travel Nurse Checklist: 12 Easy Steps

- ☐ Obtain a nursing degree
- ☐ Pass the NCLEX
- ☐ Gain 2 years of work experience
- ☐ Research & apply with travel nursing agencies to build a profile
- ☐ Obtain desired state's nursing license
- ☐ Browse & submit to job openings
- ☐ Prepare for interviews
- ☐ Review offer/contract & sign or decline
- ☐ Begin onboarding process
- ☐ Find housing & prepare to move
- ☐ Follow first day instructions for orientation
- ☐ Extend contract or repeat steps #4-11 for your next assignment

Made in the USA
Monee, IL
04 November 2026

67378316R00024